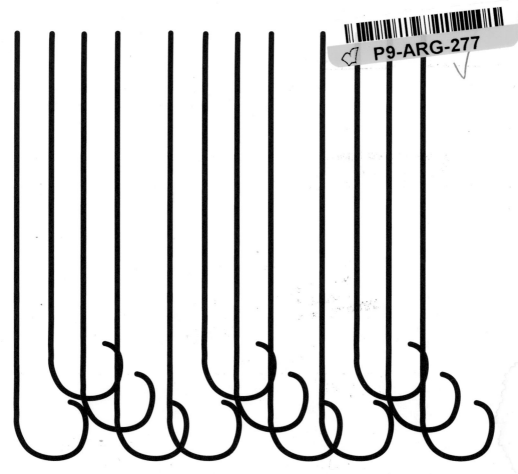

BLACK HAIR IS . . .

The <u>Complete</u> Hair Care Guide For

Today's Black Woman

By Marilyn Singleton

IMAGE PERFECT COMMUNICATIONS, INC.
Atlanta, Georgia
1992

Copyright ©1992 by Marilyn Singleton

All rights reserved including the right to reproduce this handbook or portions thereof in any form. Published by Image Perfect Communications, Inc., 1480 F Terrell Mill Rd., Suite 289, Marietta, Georgia 30067

Published in the United States of America
First Printing, 1992

Cover design and page layout: Becky Craig

Singleton, Marilyn
BLACK HAIR IS. . . The Complete Hair Care Guide For Today's Black Woman

Library of Congress Catalog Card Number 92-71170
Includes Index
ISBN 0-9632805-7-0

PUBLISHER'S NOTICE: This book is not intended to be a substitute for professional medical consultation. Nutritional and health requirements vary from person to person, depending on their general health, age, sex, weight and diet. Use this book as a reference guide only. Self-diagnosis is not advised.

ACKNOWLEDGEMENTS

An abundance of time, research and commitment are represented by the information contained within the pages of this book. I want to express my appreciation to all of the hair care specialists who contributed their knowledge, expertise and understanding of Black hair for the benefit of our readers.

For the invaluable information on hair care, health, maintenance and grooming, a very special word of appreciation is extended to dermatologists: Gloria Campbell-D'Hue, M.D., Steven S. Thomas, M.D. and Wesley S. Wilborn, M.D.

Dr. Gloria Campbell-D'Hue attended medical school at Emory University. She is an Associate of the American Academy of Dermatology and is currently in private practice in Atlanta, Georgia.

Dr. Steven S. Thomas attended medical school at the University of Illinois. His specialty training in dermatology was completed at Emory University. He is certified by the American Board of Dermatology and is a Clinical Assistant Professor at Emory University. He is presently in private practice in Decatur, Georgia.

Dr. Wesley S. Wilborn attended medical school at Maharry Medical College in Nashville, TN. He is certified by the American Board of Dermatology and is a Fellow of the American Academy of Dermatology. Dr. Wilborn is a Clinical Associate Professor of Dermatology at Emory University of Medicine. He is founder and president of Dermatologist's Products Ltd., and the formulator of all of the X-ceptional and Back Alive products. He is presently in private practice in Atlanta, GA.

For the magnificent cover, we thank nationally-acclaimed photographer, Darrell Lane, and for the beautiful cover design and page layout, a very special thanks to Becky Craig. For his superlative artistry in hair design, we thank premier stylist Charles Gregory, owner of Charles Gregory Salon in Atlanta, for his masterpiece cover hairstyle. For our cover girl's make-up, we thank the very talented Gwyniss Mosby. And, of course, thanks to our cover girl, Carole McCoy.

Special thanks to all of the hair designers who contributed their hairstyles for presentation in this book, including: Elham Awad for Uptown Hair Design Studios, Pittsburgh, PA; David Fields for DAWEED's Hair Design, Decatur, GA; Charles Gregory for Charles Gregory Salon, Atlanta, GA; Geri Mataya for Uptown Hair Design Studio, Pittsburgh, PA; Rudy Townsel for Rudy Townsel & Associates Hair Design, New York, NY, and Izear Winfrey for Uptown Hair Design Studio, Pittsburgh, PA.

The beautiful images that are seen throughout this book were captured by photographers: Archie Carpenter, Pittsburgh PA; Reggie Parker, Atlanta, GA; Bill Suttle, Pittsburgh, PA; Matthew Smith, New York, NY, and Drew Yenchak, Pittsburgh, PA.

We offer thanks to the following Makeup Artists: Sam Fine for Rudy Townsel & Associates, New York, NY; Charles Gregory for DAWEED's HAIR DESIGN, Decatur, GA; Beth Yenchak for Uptown Hair Design Studio, Pittsburgh, PA, and Izear Winfrey for Uptown Hair Design Studio, Pittsburgh, PA.

CONTENTS

iv

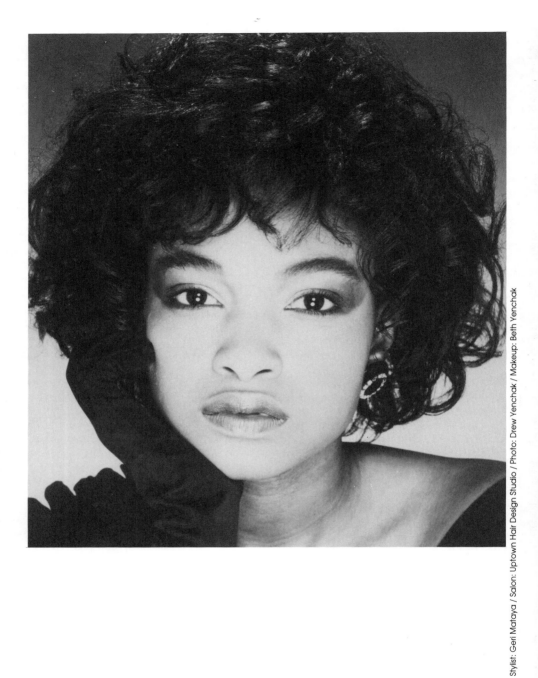

Stylist: Geri Mataya / Salon: Uptown Hair Design Studio / Photo: Drew Yenchak / Makeup: Beth Yenchak

Sweet Seduction

Preface

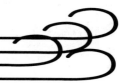

CELEBRATION OF SELF

Here we are in the second year of a new decade — the '90s. Times have changed, and so have we. We've come a long way, and it's time to celebrate. We need not celebrate a new year, nor a new decade, but rather let us celebrate ourselves! And what better way to celebrate than by becoming the very best that we can be. And what better place to start than at the very top — with our hair. *OUR HAIR* — the single most unique form of self-expression and individualized beauty.

Beautiful, healthy hair is just within reach. Finally! There is a handbook designed with you, the Black woman, in mind. This book contains facts that have been proven to assist in the promotion of hair growth and health. Your hair is your crown and glory, but beautiful hair doesn't just happen. YOU HAVE TO MAKE IT HAPPEN! The tips in this book will help take your hair to its glorious best. When your hair looks great, it sends a message to the world. It says that you are in charge of your life and have a strong sense of self.

Formulas, tonics, hair greases and other topical "miracle" potions will *not* make your hair grow. You must start from the inside out. BEAUTY STARTS FROM WITHIN... This book will give you succinct and concise instructions and guidance on how to obtain the longer, healthier, more beautiful hair you have always desired. Anybody and everybody can have beautiful hair. All it takes is commitment. Contained within these pages are tips that will most assuredly turn you into the MANE ATTRACTION at any event!

Whether your objective is to grow longer hair, or simply to have the most beautiful hair possible, this book will point you in the right direction. The rest is up to you. COMMITMENT. . . That's all it takes.

So, ladies, break out your finest crystal champagne flutes, and let the Dom Perignon flow. By the time you have completed this book, you will have plenty to celebrate. You'll be celebrating a new and improved you... A you that radiates an omnipotent expression of positive self-image. HERE'S TO HAIR! Beautiful Hair! Your Hair! Hair that will make the world stop on a dime to get a second look at you. Here's to you and new beginnings.

CHAPTER 1: Hair, What Is It Anyway?

Let's start at the beginning. What exactly is hair? Very simply, the lovely, lively tresses that frame your face are in actuality quite dead. Below the scalp surface lies the only living and reproducing area of the hair - the root. It is located at the base of each hair follicle. Hair is comprised of 97 percent protein in the form of keratin. The remaining contents are amino acids and other trace minerals. Because hair is dead matter, it cannot repair itself. The damage that you do to it, through improper handling, poor diet and excessive use and abuse of heat appliances, can be irreversible. It is, therefore, advantageous to avoid damage through a well-thought out health and beauty regimen. An ounce of prevention can be worth inches of hair.

There are three different types of hair shapes: curly/kinky, straight and wavy. The type of hair you will have is predetermined by the shape of your follicle. Curly/kinky hair grows from a flat follicle. Straight hair grows from a round follicle. Wavy hair grows from an oval follicle.

THE HAIR SHAFT

Each shaft of hair is comprised of three distinct layers: the cuticle, the cortex and the medulla.The cuticle is the outermost layer. The tough cellular formation of the cuticle resembles roof shingles. Its well-being is essential because it serves as a barrier, preventing excessive evaporation of moisture from the cortex. Moisture is vital to the elasticity of the hair. The cuticle protects the cortex from splitting.

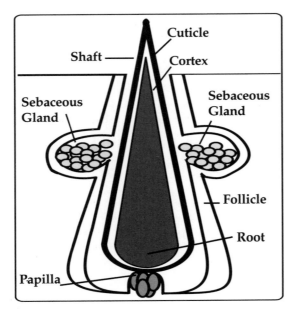

The second distinct layer is the cortex. The cortex is located directly below the cuticle and is responsible for determining the color of hair, by providing the pigment (melanin). The innermost core of the hair shaft is the medulla. The complete function of this layer is still unknown. Scientists have determined that it is present in some strands of hair, while absent in others.

CHAPTER 2: Hair Growth

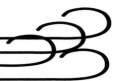

Hair grows at the rate of one-half inch per month on average. Remember, this is an average. Some people's hair will grow faster; others slower. Many Black women complain that their hair just won't grow. This simply is not true. Everybody's hair grows, but because Black hair is fragile hair, it is also more susceptible to breakage. Our hair often breaks off before we can actualize growth, which is why we must learn to handle our hair gently. The daily commitment that you make to your hair will directly affect the condition of your hair. Everything that you do and do not do will affect your hair — one way or the other. Once you understand the dynamics of your hair and the things that will adversely affect it, you will be on the road to achieving the wonderful head of hair you have always dreamed of having.

There are several factors that determine hair growth. They are: genetics, general health, diet, age and emotional state. (Of course special circumstances, i.e., pregnancy, surgery, anemia and other illnessess will also affect hair growth and loss.)

Heredity directly influences the color and texture of your hair, while your daily diet and general physical state influence its strength, health and condition. You have taken the first step to positively improving your hair by reading this handbook. The second step is to follow the advice contained within these pages, as well as advice given to you by the hair care specialist of your choice.

HOW YOUR HAIR GROWS — THREE CYCLES OF GROWTH

Hair growth is cyclical. There are three continuous cycles: anagen, catagen and telogen. The anagen cycle is the cycle of great activity. Eighty to ninety percent of your hair is growing in this cycle. Follicle activity is accelerated, contributing to the elongating of the hair shaft. This cycle can last between three to ten years.

The second cycle, catagen, is a transitional period. The follicle activity ceases. This stage can last anywhere from one to three weeks.

And finally, the third cycle, telogen, is the resting period. The follicle shrinks, hair loosens and falls out. This stage can last between three to five months. Ten to twenty percent of your hair is in a stage of rest at one time. Circumstances, such as, poor diet, surgery, anemia, etc., can prolong the telogen cycle, causing hair growth to slow down or stop completely.

NORMAL HAIR LOSS

Summer months bring about accelerated hair growth, while autumn months tend to bring about hair loss. On average, human beings lose approximately fifty to two hundred strands of hair on a daily basis. This is normal and nothing to be concerned about. Hair is constantly regenerating itself as it falls. Everybody loses hair—everyday! If, however, you notice an exorbitant or abnormal amount of hair loss, you should consult with a dermatologist or trichologist to determine the cause and possible solution. Hair loss can be symptomatic of a more serious health problem. Take no chances.

HAIR VOLUME

The number of hairs on your head is predetermined at birth by the number of hair follicles you have. The average number of hairs on the human head is 100,000. The color of your hair is a direct determinant. People with black hair have approximately 108,000 hairs on their head; brown hair is 110,000. Blonds have more follicles, averaging at the higher end of the spectrum, with approximately 140,000 hairs. Redheads have fewer follicles, averaging at the lower end of the spectrum, with approximately 90,000 hairs. There isn't anything that you can do to increase the number of hair strands on your head, but there is a variety of things that you can do to "pump up the volume" of the strands of hair you already have.

CREATING VOLUME FOR THIN HAIR

Creating the illusion of thicker hair is easier today than ever! There is a wide selection of hairstyling products on the market that will give your hair the luxurious body and volume you desire. The latest mousse innovations are designed to target specific hair types. they are lighter in weight and contain rich emollients. While mousses were originally conceived as a styling aid that would give your hair "staying power", the newer mousses are formulated to add body to hair, as they moisturize and condition. Some mousses even offer color. Spray a bit of the mousse into the palm of your hand,and apply only on roots to create the illusion of volume. Try using shampoos with special polymers, or products containing hydrolyzed protein. Hydrolyzed protein has properties that will result in temporary thickening of hair by binding to hairshafts.

If your hair is thin, and you've been contemplating making a change in your hair color, you can accomplish both objectives with one process. Hair dye actually swells the hair shaft, giving your hair glorious volume...Henna, a vegetable dye, also has thickening properties, but it is not advised for everyone. Henna can be very drying and tends to work best on untreated hair. (Refer to Chapter 16: To Dye or Not To Dye.) While you're getting a "new color attitude", you might consider an expert cut. Shorter hairstyles give thin hair a fuller appearance.

With all these wonderful hair care products and techniques at your fingertips, and a little sleight of hand, magical illusions of body and volume can be created easily.

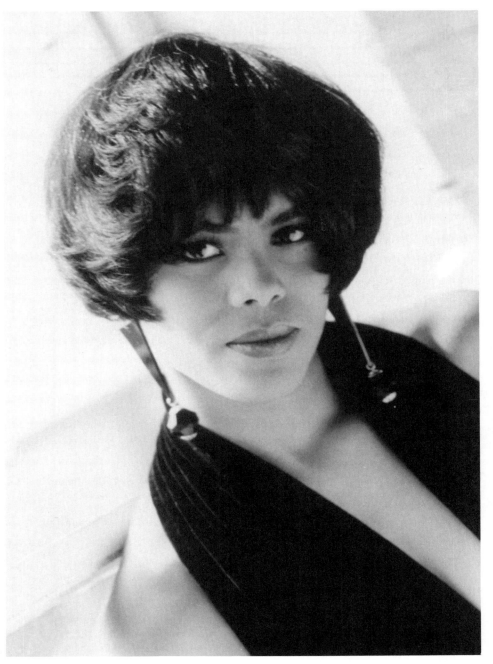

Stylist: David Fields / Salon: DAWEED'S HAIR SALON / Photo: Reggie Parker / Makeup: Charles Gregory / Model: Veronica

Bounce, Body, Volume. . .

CHAPTER 3: Beauty Starts From Within

Healthy hair requires a healthy diet. It's as simple as that! Step one in your program to establish longer, more beautiful hair is to first establish a well-balanced diet. Your diet will affect (positively or negatively) the rate at which your hair will grow. Nurture your hair by feeding the scalp the appropriate portions of essential nutrients, vitamins and minerals. Make sure that you are getting an array of foods from the Basic Four Group that we all learned about in elementary school. Avoid sugar and salt. Too much of either will wreak havoc on your hair, as well as your general health.

GETTING BACK TO THE BASICS...

I. **MEAT/POULTRY/FISH:** Two servings daily will suffice. Make sure the meat is a lean cut. Trim the skin off poultry.

II. **VEGETABLES/FRUITS:** Have a minimum of two pieces of fresh fruit daily, and one or two servings of fresh vegetables, preferably raw or slightly steamed. Cooking robs vegetables of their precious nutrients.

ALSO: Treat yourself to a green salad. Your hair will love you for it. Your body loves crunchables! While salads are great for you and your hair, oil-rich, fattening salad dressings are not. You might want to try one of the reduced-calorie varieties available in your supermarket. Read the label carefully. Instead of pouring the dressing over your salad, as is traditional, dip a forkful of salad (ever-so-gingerly) in a small bowl of dressing. You will be amazed at how little dressing you will use with this technique.

III. **DAIRY:** Avoid whole milk. Try skim or low-fat milk, instead. Yogurts, cheese (low-fat) and cottage cheese are also sources of dairy. Watch the fat contents in dairy products. While your body needs fat, too much fat is not good for your general health, weight, skin or hair. They're making perfectly suitable low-fat products now. Try them. Many of them are actually quite good and comparable in taste to the more fat-laden varieties.

IV. **CEREALS/GRAIN/BREAD/PASTA:** A small portion of this food group is essential everyday. Pasta is an excellent diet food, contrary to popular belief. Of course anything done in extravagance will be to your detriment. *MODERATION IS THE KEY TO EVERYTHING!*

While you should get your nutritional requirements from a well-balanced diet, sometimes vitamin and mineral supplements are necessary. With today's hectic lifestyles, supplements can ensure that your body is getting the tender loving care (via proper nutrients) that it deserves. To ensure that you don't overdose or become dependent on supplements, consult with a nutritionist or physician. S/he will help you establish a diet (with or without supplements) that will not exceed the RDA (Recommended Daily Allowance). RDA determines the normal amount of nutrients necessary for good health.

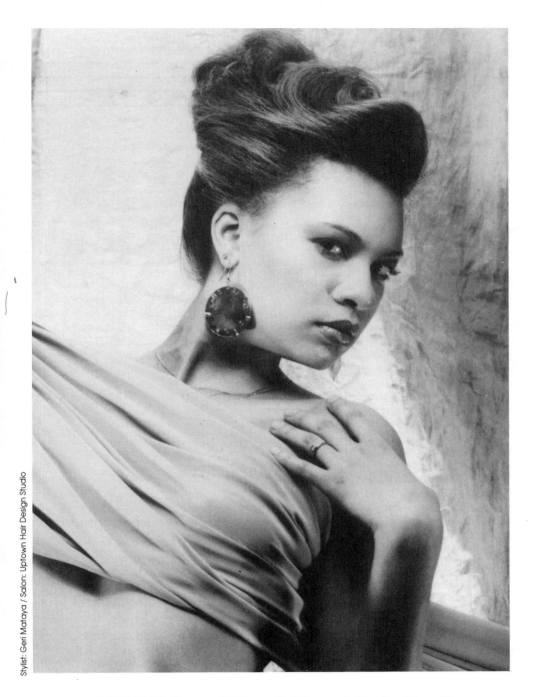

A Well-Balanced Diet...It Does A Body Good!

CHAPTER 4: Food, Vitamins and Minerals That Stimulate Hair Growth

For general good health, your diet must include a proper balance of vitamins, minerals, proteins, carbohydrates, fats and water. Now that we have established that it takes a well-balanced diet to achieve longer, healthier, more beautiful hair, let's look at some of the vitamins, minerals and nutrients that play an active role in stimulating hair growth. If you plan to incorporate vitamin and mineral supplements into your dietary regimen, be careful of the dosage consumed. Observe the RDA specifications.

VITAMIN A

There are two primary forms of vitamins: water soluble and fat soluble. With the exception of B-6, Vitamin B Complex and Vitamin C are water soluble. Your body does not store these vitamins. What your body cannot use, it will eliminate. It is therefore necessary for you to replenish these vitamins on a daily basis. On the other hand, excessive dosage of the fat soluble vitamins A, D, E and K can have devastating consequences. Your body will store fat soluble vitamins. An excessive intake can be toxic. For example, an overdose of Vitamin A can result in hair loss, dry skin, birth defects, headaches and a variety of other complications. There really is such a thing as "too much of a good thing". Because of the possible toxicity of Vitamin A, it is recommended that you get this vitamin through food sources, rather than supplements, unless otherwise advised by your physician. VITAMIN A IS ESSENTIAL TO HEALTHY HAIR! Excellent sources of Vitamin A are: beef liver, spinach, sweet potatoes, broccoli, tomatoes, collard greens, carrots, cantaloupes, etc...

VITAMIN E

Vitamin E helps circulation throughout the body, as well as to the scalp. This vitamin will help to prevent dry hair, heals dry skin and retards cellular aging. There is still controversy regarding all of the contributions Vitamin E makes to good health. Research in this area is ongoing.... Excellent food sources of Vitamin E are: wheat germ, sunflower seeds, pecans and other nuts.

PROTEIN

Your hair is 97 percent protein in a keratin form. The body does not store protein, however. It is therefore necessary for you to supply your body with the protein it needs on a daily basis. Protein is necessary for the growth and repair of cells. IT IS ESSENTIAL FOR HAIR GROWTH AND REGENERATION! On an average, .42 grams of protein (per pound of body weight) daily will suffice. For example, if you weigh 100 pounds, 42 grams of protein will approximate your daily requirement. Excellent food sources of protein are: lean cuts of meat, fish and poultry.

THE VITAMIN B GROUP

Many nutritionists and hair care specialists call The B Group, the "hair vitamins."

The B Group stimulates activity within the follicles and cells. These vitamins must be taken with a sufficient amount of protein to ensure their efficacy. A lack of the Vitamin B Group will result in hair breakage, thinning and discoloration. The B Group should be taken in the Vitamin B Complex form. Taking megadoses of one of the Vitamin B Group can result in a deficiency in one of the others.

VITAMIN B GROUP: Food Sources

• BREWER'S YEAST: I personally swear by brewer's yeast. It's an excellent source of Vitamin B complex, with the added bonus of being an excellent source of fiber... Nothing is a panacea, but I wouldn't miss a day without taking three heaping tablespoons of yeast in a glass of orange juice or tomato juice. It has done wonders for _my_ hair! It is also available in tablet form.

• WHEAT GERM: A tablespoon or two of wheat germ sprinkled over a bowl of hot porridge with a dash of raisins makes for a most nutritious breakfast. Add a slice of whole wheat toast (skip the butter), a glass of skim milk, and you have the makings of a wonderful day. Raisins are excellent sources of iron, which your hair just absolutely adores!

• Lecithin, sunflower seeds (preferably raw and unsalted), soybeans, mushrooms, green vegetables, poultry, lean meats, liver, dried beans. (Leave the fatback and ham hocks out of the bean pot. Try smoked turkey wings, if you must season with a meat.)

IRON

Iron is an essential mineral to your general body functioning. An insufficient intake of this vital mineral can result in anemia, hair loss and brittle nails. Iron's contribution to the health and beauty of your hair, skin and nails is extremely important.

Your scalp thrives on oxygen, and iron plays a major role in delivering oxygen to your scalp. Oxygen is your hair's life source. Because women lose iron during their menstruation, it is important to monitor the intake of this mineral closely. The RDA requirement for women between the ages of nineteen and fifty is 18 milligrams; ten milligrams for women fifty-one and older. There are, however, exceptions. Women who are pregnant, nursing, vegetarians or dieting should consult a physician to develop a dietary regimen that will meet their special needs. Excellent food sources for iron are: beef liver, kidney, organ meats, raisins, currants, poultry, asparagus, venison, egg yolk, shellfish, etc....

ZINC

Zinc is also one of the sixteen minerals identified as essential to good health. This mineral assists in the maintenance of healthy hair, scalp, skin and nails. Excellent food sources for zinc are: liver, turkey, lean beef, pumpkin seeds, etc...

WATER

Every cell in your body is comprised of <u>water</u>. Sufficient intake of water is absolutely essential for the healthy well-being of your entire body. Water flushes away toxic waste, curbs over-ambitious appetites, assists the metabolic processes and regulates body temperature. Every part of your body will function better when you drink adequate amounts of water. Drink at least eight glasses of water daily. The water in your tea, coffee, soft drinks and other beverages doesn't count. You can, however, consume lots of fresh fruit and vegetables to help you reach your daily water quota. Watermelons, cantaloupes, tomatoes, peaches, asparagus and various berries are a few of the fruits and vegtables that will help you accomplish your goal. These fruits and vegetables contain at least 80 percent water. You will see a vast improvement in the condition of your hair, skin, nails, eyes and body weight maintenance. So, drink up!!!

THE CHALLENGE

You spend hundreds of dollars going to the hair salon for <u>instant gratification</u>. You have your hair permed, relaxed, straightened, curled, braided, dyed, frosted, bonded and weaved. Why not really do yourself a favor and get <u>permanent gratification</u> by allocating a small amount of your hair salon dollars for a consultation with a dermatologist, nutritionist or physician. It will be the best money you have ever spent. The results will be lasting.

Beauty starts from the inside, and works its way to the outside. The bonus you will derive from taking care of your hair through a well-balanced diet and exercise is that <u>everything</u> will begin to look good: your hair, your skin, your body, your nails. You will be filled with vim, vigor and fire. You will look in the mirror and smile at the reflection that looks back at you. You'll be ready for the world, and the world will be waiting for you with open arms.

10

CHAPTER 5: Dieting And Your Hair

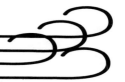

"THIN IS IN". Unfortunately, too many women fall prey to this line of thinking and will surrender any and everything (including their health) to obtain the sleek, svelte lines of the models they see adorning the covers of their favorite fashion magazines. The plain, simple truth of the matter is that every woman is not meant to be a size six. As a matter of fact, the vast majority of women wear sizes ten to fourteen. The maddening desire for women to achieve pencil-like figures has pushed many women into a constant "diet frenzy," trying each and every fad diet that becomes the rage of the moment, gaining and losing weight erratically. It's called the yo-yo syndrome.

Serious eating disorders (i.e., bulimia and anorexia nervosia) can evolve from these unnatural and undisciplined eating habits, creating the possibility for an even greater health problem —DEATH!

When you neglect the nutritional needs of your body, you also neglect the nutritional needs of your hair.

The most important thing to remember is to do everything in moderation. When dieting to lose weight, a physician should be consulted to assist you in formulating a diet low in calories and fat, while maintaining the necessary nutritional balance that your body needs to sustain it in a healthy way. Starving yourself would only be a temporary solution. Behavior-modification is a more lasting solution. Developing a well-balanced dietary regimen that suits your lifestyle (and most importantly, that you can live with comfortably) will result in healthy, permanent weight loss. Do not neglect physical exercise. A half-hour of daily (or every other day) exercise is a prerequisite to a healthy state of being. The bonus is accelerated hair growth. The heat generated from your body during exercise will speed up the rate of hair growth. And that's a fact!

CHAPTER 6: Fragile When Wet. . . Shampoo

Black hair requires shampooing approximately every five days to remove sebum (oil), dead cells and debris from hair and scalp . If hair is worn in its natural state, hair should be shampooed a <u>minimum</u> of twice a week. Use an oil-based conditioner on natural hair. Frequent shampooing allows the scalp to breathe freely; thereby, promoting hair growth. It is also beneficial in discouraging infections and stimulating the scalp.

Where you live and your lifestyle should, however, be the ultimate gauge for determining the frequency in which you shampoo and condition your hair. While Lisa, who leads a sedentary lifestyle in Selma, might only require a shampoo every seven days; Melinda, who lives in New York City, and jogs four miles daily, might require a shampoo every four or five days. At the minimum, hair should be shampooed every seven days.

If you live in a large metropolis (i.e., New York, Los Angeles, Chicago) your hair will naturally be exposed to environmental pollutants, such as automobile exhaust fumes, smog, dirt and grime. Because of these critical factors, you will need to shampoo your hair with greater frequency. Act accordingly!

Other determinants that must be factored into the shampoo frequency equation are: physical exercise (as exemplified in the case scenario previously outlined) weather and hair type. Because of the fragility of our hair, we need to minimize unnecessary encounters with our hair— especially when it is at its most fragile — wet.

If you exercise often, the perspiration build-up on your hair and scalp can render your hair unmanageable and, alas, odorous. Perspiration is quite destructive to hair. After you have engaged in strenuous exercise or sports, you should shampoo your hair as soon as possible. Perspiration will fade colored hair and deplete chemically-treated hair of its natural moisture, leaving it dry and dull in appearance. If possible, pre-condition your hair before participating in an exercise program or sports, and shampoo your hair frequently. "Perspiration has a tendency to strip, dry and make hair brittle and susceptible to breakage," says Steven Thomas, M.D., a dermatologist.

Hot, sticky and humid summer weather will also affect your hair adversely. No one knows better than you, when your hair needs to be shampooed. Its performance, manageability, sheen and general appearance are dead giveaways. If that's not enough of a clue, the mere combing of your hair should provide the conclusive tell-tale sign that the time has arrived for a shampoo. The accumulation of exfoliated skin cells and sebum build-up will result in flaking. Don't put off shampooing your hair. Shampoo it, when it is time.

When using hair type as a barometer for determining the frequency of shampooing, common sense should prevail. Hair type is determined by how much sebum is produced by your sebaceous glands. These glands open into the hair follicle. Naturally, a very active sebaceous gland will result in oily hair; less active — dry, and normal will fall somewhere in the middle. Obviously, oily hair will need to be shampooed with greater frequency than dry hair.

• **<u>NORMAL HAIR</u>:** This is the easiest hair type to take care of. It is generally soft and manageable. The amount of oil and moisture in normal hair sufficiently minimizes breakage, and coats the hair shaft to protect against loss of natural moisture.

RECOMMENDATION: Use a PH-balanced shampoo. (The term PH-balance sounds scientific/mysterious/technical. In actuality, it is a very simple concept... A PH7 contains a neutral acid/alkaline content. Anything lower than PH7 has a high acidity level; anything higher than PH7 has a high alkaline level.) Follow-through with an instant, moisturizing conditioner. You might want to use a deep-penetrating conditioner once-a-month. RINSE HAIR THOROUGHLY!

• **<u>DRY HAIR</u>:** This type of hair lacks moisture and oils. There is a low level of sebum and excessive moisture loss from hair shafts. Dry hair is characterized as dull, lackluster and lacking elasticity. It is frequently plagued with split ends. (See Chapter 14, The Hair Trim & Split Ends.) Dry hair can be a result of over-processing, neglect or maturity. As we age, the production of sebum decreases. Dry hair can also occur naturally. Keep styles simple. <u>Do</u> use a lightweight hairdressing or emulsion. Apply directly to hair, not scalp! Avoid salt!

RECOMMENDATION: Use a mild, PH-balanced shampoo. Follow-through with a deep-penetrating conditioner, rich in emollients and moisturizers. (Avoid conditioners containing balsam.) RINSE HAIR THOROUGHLY! If you must use a hair dryer or blow dryer, take more time and lower the temperature to a cooler setting. Trim ends approximately every six weeks to minimize breakage and eliminate split ends. Do *not* use oils, greases and pomades on the scalp directly. Contrary to popular belief, oiling the scalp does not encourage hair growth. Dermatologists, trichologists and other hair care specialists, categorically, refute this myth. Oiling the scalp will impede hair growth by suffocating and clogging hair follicles. Allow your hair follicles to breathe. In addition to deterring hair growth, oiling the scalp can result in dandruff, temple acne, weigh down hair, and the oil can act as a magnet to environmental pollutants. Opt instead, for an oil-free, clean, healthy scalp that breathes. A breathing scalp will accelerate and encourage hair growth.

• **<u>OILY HAIR</u>:** This is greasy hair that needs to be shampooed frequently. If not, it will weigh itself down and just lie there. Oily hair is caused by excessive production of sebum.

RECOMMENDATION: Use a PH-balanced, cleansing shampoo. Follow-through with an oil-free, instant conditioner. Concentrate the conditioner on the tips of your hair. RINSE THOROUGHLY! Do not use oils, greases or pomades.

• **DAMAGED HAIR**: Hair that is damaged, like all types of hair, should be treated gently. Add an extra dose of TLC to this type of hair. It is extremely fragile. Damaged hair is usually over-processed, dry, brittle hair, prone to breakage and splits at the slightest provocation. SO DON'T PROVOKE IT!

RECOMMENDATION: Use a low PH-balanced shampoo. Follow through with a deep-penetrating, moisturizing conditioner. RINSE THOROUGHLY! If you must use a hair dryer or blow dryer, lower the temperature to a cooler setting. Use a diffuser on your blow dryer. Keep your hairstyles simple. A trim every six weeks will help you control dry, split ends.

Black hair is extremely fragile when wet, so proceed with extreme caution to avoid unnecessary breakage. Use a PH-balanced, diluted shampoo, specifically formulated for your hair type. Consult with your hairstylist for guidance in selecting the best shampoo and conditioner for your hair type and specific hair problems. You might want to use the identical products that are used in your beauty salon. Many beauty parlors sell these products as an auxiliary business.

Once you have selected the shampoo and conditioner that's right for you, make sure that you rinse your hair thoroughly. This is indeed very important. Shampoo and conditioner build-up is the primary cause for dull, lackluster hair. Start out with tepid water, gradually making the water cooler. A cool final rinse will smooth hair cuticles, shrink hair shafts, and give your hair a shiny and healthy appearance.

CHAPTER 7: The Conditioner And Moisturizer

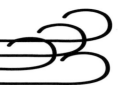

Conditioners and moisturizers should be applied to clean hair. They should be applied directly to the hair, not the scalp. Leave the conditioner on hair the prescribed amount of time outlined in the directions on the bottle label. Because Black hair tends to tangle easily, it is necessary to condition the hair every time you shampoo to make the hair more manageable and to protect it from damage. The conditioner should be concentrated on tips of hair, where damage, breakage and split ends occur most frequently.

The heat appliances and chemical processes used by Black women deplete their hair of its natural moisture. In order to maintain, replace or improve moisture levels and elasticity, it is absolutely imperative that Black women condition their hair regularly. Deep-penetrating conditioners should be used approximately every other week on hair that has been severely abused or is excessively dry.

WHAT A CONDITIONER WILL DO FOR YOUR HAIR

In addition to detangling hair (rendering it more manageable), a conditioner will give hair a sleeker, healthier appearance. The conditioner coats the hair shaft, causing the cuticles to lie flat, enabling it to reflect light. The hair appears shinier. It also serves as a protectant to the cuticles and hair shafts, while sealing in moisture.

HAIR PRODUCTS: THE INGREDIENTS TO LOOK FOR

Look for products containing jojoba oils, silk proteins, camomile, panthenol, aloe vera and rosewater. These ingredients have conditioning properties. Avoid balsams and alcohol. Balsams simply do not provide the much- needed moisture that Black hair requires for maximum health, and alcohol is very drying. Make it a habit to read the label of your hair care products before making a purchase. The ingredients appear according to their proportional dominance in the product. For example, water is usually the first ingredient listed on shampoo labels.

FRAGILE WHEN WET

HANDLE WITH CARE FACT SHEET

1.Instead of rubbing your hair vigorously with a towel to get it dry, wrap the towel (Turkish-style) around your head, and blot ever-so gently to remove excess water.

2. Absolutely never use a brush on your fragile hair when it is wet. Hair breakage will most assuredly be a consequence.

3. <u>Do</u> use a wide-toothed, saw-cut comb to remove snarls and tangles....Hard rubber or tortoise shell is your best bet.

4. Blow dry your hair on the lower temperature setting. If using a hair dryer, the same rule applies.

5. Hold blow dryer at least six inches from your head, rotating the dryer around your head frequently. Direct heat is extremely damaging.

6. Comb hair from the ends, working your way gently up to the roots.

7. **NEVER USE SPONGE OR BRUSH ROLLERS!**

8. Before applying curling irons to your hair, make sure that your hair is completely dry.

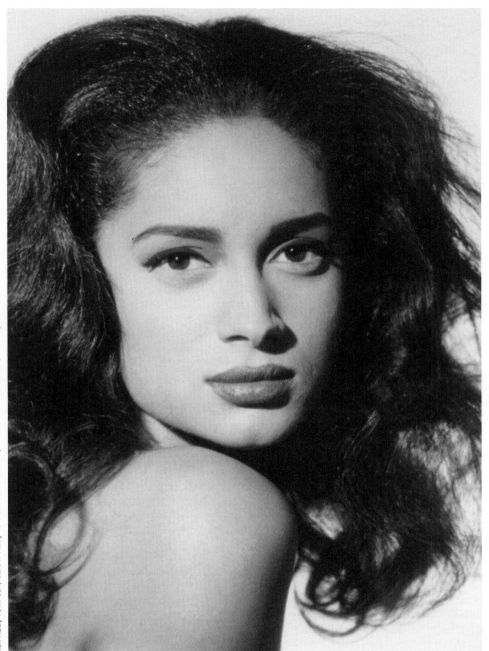

Hair Styling and Profiling

CHAPTER 8: The Hairset

After you have shampooed and conditioned your hair, the next step is to decide on a hairstyle. The manner you choose to set your hair will influence the curl, flow, bounce and volume of your hairstyle. You can choose a variety of methods of achieving the curl that you desire: roller set, pin curl, wrap , etc. Choosing the correct set, roller and rolling technique are crucial ingredients in obtaining your hairstyling goals.

THE HAIR ROLLER SET

Section and part the piece of hair that is to be rolled. Section off only as much hair as your roller will accommodate easily. For larger, free flowing curls, use bigger hair rollers. For a tighter, longer-lasting curl, use smaller rollers. Lift sectioned piece of hair from the scalp to its full length. Apply setting lotion and comb through. Catch ends of hair with end papers. Make sure that you use end papers on all hair that you plan to roll to ensure a smoother set. Wind hair around roller. Insert plastic stick. Sit under hair dryer that has been set on a low temperature, until hair is completely dry. Plastic, wire mesh or Velcro rollers work best. Velcro and mesh rollers allow the hair to dry quickly and breathe freely, without depleting its natural moisture level.

The "BIG DON'Ts" in hair roller sets are:

(1) DON'T SLEEP IN HAIR ROLLERS — EVER!

(2) DON'T USE SPONGE OR BRUSH ROLLERS — EVER!

THE PIN CURL

Uniformity is key. Each curl should have the same amount of hair. Bobby pins tend to leave a large number of impressions in the hair when they are removed. To avoid this dilemma, use hair clips. To achieve a professional curl using this method, ask your hairstylist to demonstrate the proper technique of winding and pinning the hair in place.

An alternative method of pin curling is the barrel curl. You simply section hair, curl and pin. If you want loose curls, make the sections larger; tighter curls, make the sections smaller. Extend each section to its fullest length, and use you finger to curl hair into the shape of a roller. Roll hair in the direction that your style requires. Place two bobby pins inside the bottom of the curl, securing at the scalp. In the morning, you will have a beautiful set, with minimum trauma to your hair.

THE WRAP

The wrap is one of the more exciting hair setting innovations of recent times. Simply use your head as a roller, and wrap hair smoothly around it. This method produces some of the more classic hairstyles, i.e, pageboy, china doll, etc.

CHAPTER 9: Tools Of The Trade

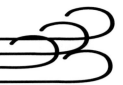

BLOW DRYERS AND HAIR DRYERS

Total avoidance of blow dryers and hair dryers is virtually impossible for most of today's on-the-go women, nor would we want to have to go back to the Stone Ages just to maintain healthy, beautiful hair. Fortunately, abstinence is not necessary. The time-saving advantages offered by these appliances can never be denied, but *moderation* is essential. Daily (or constant) use of either one of these appliances will, most assuredly, strip hair of its natural oils and moisture, resulting in dull, brittle hair. Excessive heat can also trigger accelerated activity in the sebaceous glands, resulting in an oily scalp.

THE BLOW DRYER

When blow drying your hair, set the temperature to medium. Keep the blow dryer at least six inches from your hair. Select a dryer with a wide nozzle to help diffuse the heat. I know it's tempting to put the setting on "hot" to expedite the drying process, but the inevitable damage that will result from this unbridled, concentrated heat is simply not worth the few minutes you save. Take a little extra time. Massive horsepower is also not necessary. A blow dryer with 1000 watts or less will suffice and will be less expensive than one with greater wattage. Keep your hand moving. Don't stay on one section of hair for too long. A few seconds will do it. Start at the nape and work up to the crown. Be kind to your hair.

THE HAIR DRYER

There are two types of hair dryers that are most commonly manufactured for home usage. The soft bonnet variety or the hard hood. The latter resembles the type used in professional hair salons. I personally prefer the soft bonnet variety, because it allows greater mobility. With an extension cord, I have full access to all of the rooms of my home, and I am able to complete household chores or business-related assignments, while simultaneously drying my hair. This extra bonus of flexibility makes it easier for me to remain under the dryer for the longer time required when using a cool to medium setting, which is absolutely imperative. Once again, the hot temperature setting is damaging to the hair. 1,200 watts and under is an adequate amount of power.

THE BRUSH

Keep brushing to a minimum, but when you must, choose a natural boar bristle or ball-tipped brush. Most dermatologists recommend the latter for Black hair. The ball-tipped brushes offer additional protection. Do not, however, detangle Black hair with any type of brush, and never brush your fragile wet hair!!! Instead, use a saw-cut, wide-toothed rubber comb. Start from the hair tips, and work your way gently towards the scalp. And remember, it makes absolutely no sense to keep your hair clean, and then to use dirty grooming tools. Keep your comb and brush clean. Everytime you shampoo your hair, wash your comb and brush. Remove strands of hair from your brush with your comb. Squeeze a tiny bit of shampoo onto the bristles of your brush. While holding your brush under running water, run your comb through it. Rinse with warm water. Repeat...Shake the excess water from your comb and brush. Place both on a towel and allow to air-dry. The bristles of your brush should be facing down.

THE HAIR COMB

The hair comb is the most frequently used hair grooming tool. Its selection should, therefore, be given great consideration. A saw-cut, wide-toothed rubber or tortoise shell comb is best. A saw-cut comb is one in which each tooth is cut into the comb. This type of comb is devoid of rough, jagged edges. Your comb must be kept clean.

THE CURLING IRON

The curling iron is a modern convenience. Unfortunately, many Black women have become enslaved to them. It's so simple to wake up in the morning, plug the irons in, and put a few quick curls in the hair. This direct heat, however, is quite damaging. I know how hard it would be for you to give up your curling irons completely, but, once again, exercise moderation and common sense. Do not use these appliances daily. You must give your hair a rest. Allow the iron to remain on each section of hair no longer than thirty seconds. Do not let the iron touch your scalp. This, obviously, can result in blistering of the scalp and permanent damage to follicles. Excessive use of curling irons can result in dry, dull and brittle hair. Be creative in juggling your methods and techniques of obtaining curls. Use some of the less damaging methods with greater frequency. Your hair will love you for it.

BOBBY PINS AND HAIRPINS

Obviously, your hairpins and bobby pins should match your hair coloring as closely as possible. When the rubber tips come off, throw your pins in the garbage — immediately! The exposed sharp tips can scratch and damage your scalp. It's not worth it! These accessories cost pennies to replace.

Also, don't pull and pin hair tightly, a la chignon, ponytails, braids, cornrows, etc... This practice can result in breakage and traction alopecia (a hair loss condition). Remove pins before you go to bed. Allow your hair to breathe and flow freely.

RUBBER BANDS

Forget about using rubber bands as hair accessories. They are extremely damaging. They cut, tear and rip the hair. Instead, opt for coated elastic ponytail holders, which can be purchased inexpensively. Remove before retiring to bed.

THE SATIN PILLOWCASE

Treat yourself to a satin or silk pillowcase. Your set will last much longer, and hair breakage will be minimized.

CHAPTER 10: Improving Scalp Circulation

BRUSHING

"ONE HUNDRED BRUSH STROKES WILL MAKE YOUR HAIR SHINY AND BEAUTIFUL!" This is something that every little girl has heard and has believed. Well, it's definitely time to lay that old wives' tale to rest. Black hair is fragile hair. While brushing the hair <u>does</u> stimulate the scalp and helps to distribute oils, the devastating negative effects far outweigh whatever advantages can be derived from this archaic and damaging practice. Excessive brushing will result in split ends and hair breakage. Over-ambitious brushing can uproot hairs in the telogen stage (resting) of growth. Use a hair brush minimally. Brush only when it is absolutely necessary to obtain a particular hairstyle. When you must brush, be gentle and use a natural boar or ball-tipped bristle brush to avoid scratching and irritating the scalp. Brushes with ball-tipped bristles add extra protection and can be found in any number of health and beauty supply stores.

Carefully applied massages offer many of the advantages of brushing without the drawbacks. "My suggestion to my patients is to massage. I find that a good massage stimulates circulation, distributes oils, and is a method of relaxation," says Gloria Campbell-D'Hue, a dermatologist in Atlanta.

THE MASSAGE

The very first step of preparation in ensuring an invigorating, healthy scalp massage is to check your fingernails. Yes, that's right. YOUR FINGERNAILS! This step is critical to any hand-to-hair contact, including the shampoo. Make sure that you don't have any hang nails. Jagged or split nails can cause severe damage by getting caught up in hair and causing breakage, often from the root. So make sure that your nails are smooth before beginning.

Now that you have a well-balanced, nutritious diet, you want to make sure that all of those wonderful nutrients have maximized impact on the condition of your hair. The massage helps to deliver nutrients to the scalp. It helps to feed your hair. Proper massage will make a tight scalp pliable and enhance the health of the scalp, while accelerating and maintaining the growth of your hair.

Massage your scalp every time you shampoo and an additional once-a-week treatment for improved circulation. Use the pads of your fingers. Make sure that you *do not* use your fingernails, which will scratch and break the skin of your scalp. Place your fingers underneath the hair, firmly onto the scalp. Spread your fingers apart and gently knead with your fingers in a stationary position. Start at the temples. Work your way up to the crown of the head, and then, down to the base of the neck. A well-aplied massage should always go from front to back, following the route of blood circulation. Concentrate on one area at a time, devoting approximately a minute or two to each spot. Mmm! Doesn't that feel good?

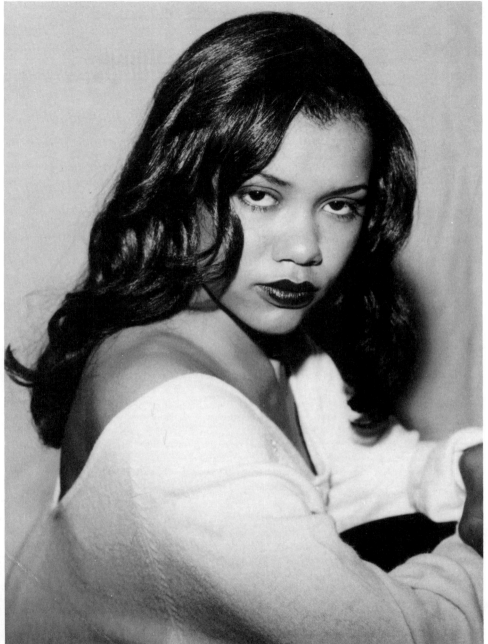

Stylist: Dwight Eubanks / Salon: Purple Door / Photo: Steven Kindred / Makeup: Naron / Model Shree Cannonier

Some Enchanted Evening. . .

CHAPTER 11: Stress And Your Tresses

More and more women are finding themselves in decision-making, wheeling and dealing, executive positions. The power is good... The money is good.... The boost to the self-esteem is good. Unfortunately, the stress that often accompanies these positions is *not* so good. Additionally, it is not only corporate big wheels who feel the pressure of the nine-to-five, work-a-day, dog-eat-dog existence in Corporate America. Working women on every level often find themselves victims of stress. Trying to juggle a career and being a wife, mother, daughter, sister, friend and lover is often a burdensome task, which can result in circuit overload, aka, stress. And stress can (and will) cause hair to fall out. One of the most common causes of alopecia areata, a hair loss condition, is stress. Round, hairless patches, devoid of scarring, are characteristic of this condition. According to Dr. Campbell-D'Hue, hair is one of the cells in our body that has a very high turnover rate. Our hair is an accurate barometer of our general health. When something goes wrong with the body, one of the first places that will be affected adversely is the hair.

While it might be difficult at first, try to allot a special "quiet time" for yourself. The time you allot for physical exercise can also be the time you devote to your mental well-being. Try yoga exercises. They are very relaxing. If you find yourself feeling particularly frazzled during the day, instead of succumbing to the pressure, stop and take a deep breath. Consciously inhale... exhale. Take a minute to recompose yourself, to release the tension. Try placing plants around the office. They help us to breathe easier, and their beauty will remind you of life's natural order. Make sure that you get six to eight hours of sleep nightly, and of course, maintain a properly balanced diet. When you have so many projects on your corporate plate, it's tempting to grab a quick bite, which usually turns out to be an oil-packed, calorie-heavy, fast food burger. Don't give in to this temptation. The price is too high to pay. If you must, brown-bag a nutritious meal. My favorite is tuna on pita bread with mushrooms, lettuce and tomatoes. I throw in a few carrot sticks and celery stalks, a fresh fruit, juice, and I'm "good to go."

TIME MANAGEMENT is critical for women who find themselves juggling a multitude of tasks. Manage your time; don't let it manage you. SAVE YOUR HEALTH AND YOUR HAIR. Take time and smell the roses!

CHAPTER 12: Problems That Plague Hair And Scalp

TRACTION ALOPECIA

Traction alopecia has been mentioned several times throughout this book. This hair loss condition is a result of undue tension placed on hair roots for a prolonged period of time. Pronounced hair loss around the temple area is quite common in traction alopecia. According to dermatologist Steven Thomas, M.D., many Black women experience this condition as a consequence of braiding, cornrowing and rolling their hair too tautly. He cites improperly fitted wigs as another problem. The remedy for traction alopecia is very simple... Simply <u>stop</u> the styling practice that has created the condition. With the cessation, hair growth should resume within several months. If these styling practices continue, **permanent alopecia can be the consequence.** HAIR <u>SHOULD</u> <u>NEVER</u> <u>BE</u> PULLED <u>TIGHTLY</u> <u>WHEN</u> <u>STYLED.</u>

Apparently Black women are beginning to get the message. Dr. Gloria Campbell-D'Hue, a dermatologist, reports that the number of Black women coming into her office with traction alopecia has decreased over the last few years.

ABNORMAL HAIR LOSS

According to dermatologist Wesley S. Wilborn, M.D., many postpartum women suffer with a hair loss condition called telogen effluvium. Physical and emotional stress brought on by surgery, high fever, chemotherapy or prescription and non-prescription drugs can also precipitate a bout of telogen effluvium. This condition causes hair to shift prematurely into the telogen stage (resting) of growth, resulting in hair loss. Once the traumatic situation has been resolved, however, the hair generally begins to regrow within several months. Dr. Wilborn advises that if you notice that your hair is breaking off at the **root**, you should consult with a dermatologist for proper diagnosis.

There are a number of hair loss conditions that arise for a variety of reasons. This book is <u>not</u> designed for self-diagnosis. If you notice an inordinate number of hairs on your pillow, in your comb or on your clothing, you should visit your dermatologist for an accurate diagnosis and corresponding treatment. A dermatologist is a medical doctor trained to diagnose and treat disease of the hair, skin and nails.

ROGAINE

Rogaine is a topical prescription drug, which contains 2 percent Minoxidil. It treats certain types of hair loss conditions. To date, reports by doctors, scientists and patients have been favorable. According to dermatologist Steven Thomas, M.D., Rogaine has been well-documented to be effective in those hair losses that are categorized as androgenetic alopecia or pattern baldness. He says, "While Rogaine is not a panacea to hair loss, it is helpful in treating certain types of alopecia, where there is a marked amount of thinning around the crown of the head. Approximately 40 to 45 percent of people, who have had Rogaine administered to them, have actualized <u>significant</u> regrowth. By significant, we mean regrowth that is noticeable to both the scientist and the patient." Rogaine has been approved by the Food and Drug Administration (F.D.A.).

Scientists have searched for centuries for a cure of baldness. While the search still continues, Rogaine does seem to offer a means of _managing_ specific types of hair loss. Rogaine is, however, expensive. If you are experiencing hair loss problems, speak with your dermatologist to find out if Rogaine is right for you.

DANDRUFF

Dandruff is a general terminology applied to a variety of scaly, flaky scalp conditions. The two most common types of dandruff are seborrhea (plain dandruff) and seborrheic dermatitis, a more severe form of dandruff. When dandruff occurs, we tend to believe that our scalps are suffering from excessive dryness. In actuality, the opposite is usually true. A scaly, flaky scalp is generally symptomatic of an _excessively_ oily scalp. Dandruff can result from an over-production of oil, subsequently causing the scalp to shed dead cells. The popular practice among Blacks of oiling the scalp to promote hair growth is a myth and must be deleted from our hair care routines. Contrary to stimulating hair growth, this practice actually retards hair growth by not allowing the hair to grow naturally. According to dermatologist Gloria Campbell-D'Hue, M.D., each hair in our scalp has its own oil gland that lubricates it. By shampooing once-a-week, the oil glands can continue to lubricate the hair, without a build-up of scalp oils and bacteria. The practice of oiling the scalp can aggravate a pre-existing condition of seborrheic dermatitis or it can trigger a new case of seborrheic dermatitis.

Research estimates that approximately 36 to 70 percent of Americans have suffered with a dandruff condition at some point in their lives. If _you_ should develop a case of dandruff, Dr. Campbell-D'Hue recommends that you follow these guidelines:

1. Wash your hair at least once-a-week. Use an antidandruff shampoo.

2. Make sure that you have a well-balanced diet.

3. Do _not_ oil your scalp. Use lightweight hair care products. If you must have a sheen, use a _spray sheen._

Dandruff can be combatted easily with consistent and persistent attention directed towards your diet, frequent shampooing and good grooming habits. Also, drink lots of water. Dermatologist Wesley S. Wilborn, M.D. recommends that his patients apply antidandruff shampoos directly to the scalp for approximately 20 minutes. A cotton ball can be used as an applicator. Rinse thoroughly, then shampoo and condition with your regular products. According to Dr. Wilborn, many of the commercial antidandruff shampoos are too harsh to apply directly to the hair. They can cause the hair to become dry and brittle. These products usually contain one or more of the following ingredients: tar, sulfur, zinc pyrithione, selenium or salicylic acid. Within four weeks you should notice an improvement. If your scalp _doesn't_ respond to the common sense regimen outlined above, visit your dermatologist for a correct diagnosis of your condition. Other conditions, such as, psoriasis, fungal infections, scalp disease and tumors can resemble dandruff. Once your doctor has identified your problem, s/he can prescribe a daily hair care regimen, diet and medications that are compatible to your specific condition.

SNAP! CRACKLE! POP! AN OUNCE OF PREVENTION...

Hair that snarls and tangles can be exasperating. Unfortunately, snarling and tangling are facts of life, resulting from improper handling and flagrant abuse and disregard of the hair. On the other side of the coin, even hair treated properly will suffer from occasional snarls and tangles. Excessively hot heat appliances, improper shampooing and conditioning and contrived hairstyles can all contribute to this problem. Snarls are inevitable when cuticles of the hair are damaged. To unsnarl dry hair, try applying a small amount of moisturizer to your hair. Using a wide-toothed, hard rubber or tortoise shell comb, work your way from the ends of your hair to the scalp. Easy does it! After shampooing, use plenty of deep-penetrating, moisturizing conditioner or reconstructor. RINSE THOROUGHLY.

THINGS TO AVOID

- Do **not** sleep in rollers.
- Do **not** mix chemicals, i.e., curl perm on top of relaxer.
- Do **not** use sponge rollers. They rob hair of precious moisture.
- Do **not** use brush rollers. They cause severe hair breakage.
- Do **not** use excessively <u>hot</u> heat appliances.Lower to a cooler setting.
- Do **not** wear rubberbands. They will cause hair breakage.
- Do **not** wear hair <u>tightly</u> pulled back or braided <u>tightly.</u>
- Do **not** wear contrived hairstyles on a daily basis. Save them for special occasions.

THINGS TO DO FOR HEALTHY HAIR

- **Do** trim your hair every six to eight weeks.
- **Do** sleep on a silk or satin pillowcase, or wrap your hair in a silky scarf before retiring. You'll rise to a new day with your hairstyle still in place, and you would have avoided hair breakage.
- **Do** use end papers when rolling your hair.
- **Do** use a thermal spray when you use heat appliances.
- **Do** condition your hair each and every time you shampoo.
- **Do** avoid hair products containing alcohol and balsam. They're drying.
- **Do** wear a silky scarf beneath your wool hats to protect your hair from breakage.
- **Do** drink plenty of water.
- **Do** exercise regularly.
- And, last but certainly not least, **do** maintain a well-balanced diet.

CHAPTER 13: Finding A Good Hairstylist

For Black women living in large metropolitan areas, finding a well-trained hair professional is a fairly simple task. By scanning fashion and beauty magazines (particularly the ones targeted to Black audiences (i.e., *Essence* and *Ebony* magazines), you will find various salons and hairstylists featured. Most often, the salons will be located in Los Angeles or New York. *Essence* magazine, however, recently did an article that featured four-star hair salons located in various parts of the nation:"Eight Great Full Service Salons Nationwide," March 1991.

If you live in a smaller city, all is not lost. The best way to find a stylist is to become an active observer of beautiful Black hair. Observe women with great hair, and then, ask them who their stylist is. Don't just stop with one woman. Ask several. You'll probably hear the name of one or two stylists from several of the women you approach. Most women will be more than willing to reveal their stylist's name to you, and will be extremely flattered that you asked, so don't be shy.

After you decide on a stylist, I would suggest that the first visit be more of a "look-see". Talk to your stylist. Tell him/her what your likes and dislikes are. Discuss your lifestyle. If you see a hairstyle in a magazine that you like, bring it along. S/he will be able to tell you if you can realistically achieve that particular style. Open the lines of communications with your very first visit....Set the pace! This can be the start of a beautiful relationship.

On your first appointment, don't get something drastic done. Test the waters first. Try a wash and set. You'll be able to determine if s/he is sensitive to your likes and dislikes, and most importantly, if s/he follows directions. If the new stylist can't get the simple things done to your satisfaction, you would have spared yourself the ordeal of a major hair catastrophe. Get to know and trust your stylist. One visit is usually all it takes to cross that bridge. Don't forget to show your appreciation with a tip that amounts to fifteen percent of the bill. Etiquette dictates "zero tip" for the salon owner, even if she styles your hair, and at least one dollar for the shampooer.

CHAPTER 14: The Hair Trim And Split Ends

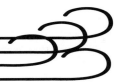

Split ends... We all get them, and they're really nothing to get overly alarmed about. There is, however, only one solution to split ends, and that is a pair of scissors. I have never seen a beautiful head of hair that was filled with split ends. The two conditions simply cannot co-exist. Split ends give hair a dull appearance.

Many Black women absolutely hate having their hair trimmed, opting instead to hang on to every precious inch of hair; no matter how damaged. Unfortunately, this attitude is counter-productive to the goal of hair growth and health. Regular trims (every six to eight weeks) are a prerequisite for establishing maximum length and beauty.

THE SCISSOR HAPPY HAIRSTYLIST!

Yes, s/he does exist. I have listened to complaints from both white and Black women, regarding stylists who take the liberty of cutting their hair into the latest hair rage, or simply cutting much more hair than requested. Once hair is cut, it's too late. Consequently, you must take your fate into your own hands. When you sit in your hairstylist's chair, you must throw your timidness out of the window. You must tell her/him what you want. I never ask for a "trim," instead I request a "snip." I expressly and directly tell my stylist not to attempt to even my hair on all sides, but rather to "snip" the split ends. The usage of the word "snip" (in lieu of trim) immediately alerts the stylist of my preference to maintain maximum length. Do *not* leave this assumption, however, to your stylist's imagination. TELL HER! Many stylists want to play Picasso or Michelangelo with your hair. Their job is to make you as beautiful as possible. A good stylist is in essence a creative artist, working her wizardry on your locks, but their definition of what makes you beautiful, and your definition might not coincide. Remember, you must live with the final product.

The stylist might take into consideration your face shape, neck length, cheekbones, height and facial features, when determining what hairstyle would be most becoming on you. Her conclusion might be that you would look great in a short hairstyle. S/he might even be right, but if you're dead set on having longer hair, you will not be happy with the cut. No matter how wonderful it is! Communications between stylist and patron is imperative in achieving mutually satisfying results. Afterall, your stylist wants your business, and s/he should be more than happy to comply with your wishes. Don't allow your stylist to impose her aesthetics on you. It's your hair, and you are, afterall, paying for her service. It does not come free. In order to achieve the results you want, work closely with your stylist. Be explicit in instructing your stylist of your wants, desires and objectives. You should work together as a team to achieve your goals. Think of your stylist as a personal consultant. Use her training to your benefit. Don't be intimidated. Once you have found a good stylist, stick with her. A good stylist can make all the difference in the world.

The bottom line is, however, that you must trim your hair regularly. If you don't trim, the consequences will be the defeat of your ultimate goal - to grow longer, healthier, more beautiful hair.

WHAT ARE SPLIT ENDS?

Split ends are simply the separation of individual hair cell layers. They result from consistent abuse to the hair. While trimming your split ends might be a temporary solution, and the only solution once they exist, behavior modification is a more permanent solution. Modify your behavior by treating your hair with gentle loving respect. It is virtually impossible to totally prevent split ends, but by treating your fragile hair with the TLC that it deserves, you can decrease the frequency of occurrence. TREAT YOUR HAIR KINDER!!!

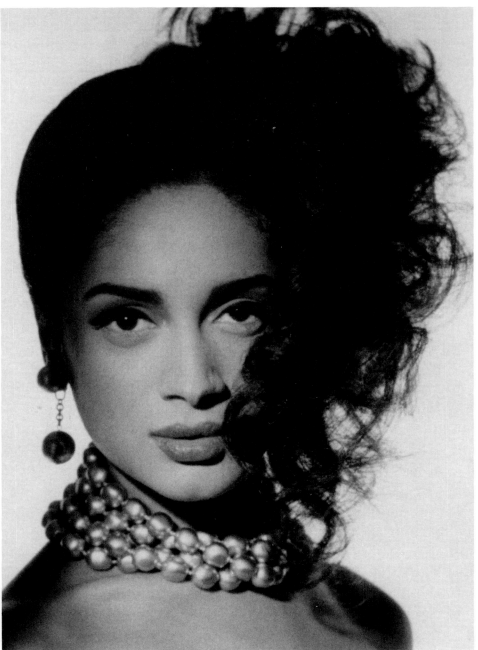

Elegance

CHAPTER 15: A Myriad Of Styling Options

Never before has the Black woman had so many styling options at her fingertips. She can have straight hair, curly hair, natural hair, twisted hair, braided hair, wavy hair and texturized hair, and she has a variety of ways to achieve these diverse looks.

If she wants to wear her hair straight, but wants the option to change her mind at whim, she can select warm comb pressing (Press and Curl). This option allows her to wear her hair in an Afro, as well. All it takes is a shampoo, and the straightened hair immediately reverts back to its natural state. If she's looking for something more permanent; something that won't be so easily affected by humidity, perspiration or water, the relaxer is a viable option. There are even new innovations that will allow her to go from straight to curly in a 24-hour period.

If she chooses to wear her hair in a variety of ways that compliment the natural texture and curl pattern of her hair (i.e., cornrowing, Afro, corkscrews), a good hair cut, shampoo, conditioning and moisturizing are the only steps necessary to achieve her objective.

THE MODIFIED PRESS AND CURL (WARM COMB STRAIGHTENING)

While the original term used by Blacks to describe the pressing process was "hot comb straightening", a _hot_ comb should never be applied to the hair. The excessive heat is drying, and will most assuredly result in breakage. The comb should be warm. The heat provided by your electric curling wand will provide the additional sleekness in style.

The disadvantage of warm comb pressing is that it only lasts from shampoo-to-shampoo. Humidity, perspiration and water will cause the hair to revert. However the advantage is that you have immeasurable versatility. You can fluctuate from straightened and curly styles to natural styles.

For decades millions of Black women straightened their hair with a hot comb. Almost a century ago (1901), the daughter of slaves, Madame C.J. Walker, used her genius and innovation to develop the metal pressing comb. Madame C.J. Walker was America's first Black millionairess. The press and curl technique of straightening and curling the hair is still quite popular today. While the technique has been modified, the press and curl still remains a viable styling option for the Black woman.

WARM COMB STRAIGHTENING— WHAT TO AVOID

• Don't use an excessively hot comb on your fragile hair. That old piece of white tissue that your mother used to determine the hotness of the comb is as viable as ever. Use it to test the degree of heat absorbed by the comb. If the comb is too hot, it will singe the tissue, or leave a brown tinge. A clean, white towel can also be used for this purpose.

• Don't apply a heated straightening comb to unclean hair. Shampoo and condition your hair prior to straightening it. Otherwise, you'll be baking the dirt and grime right into your hair.

• Don't apply a straightening comb to wet (or even slightly damp) hair. Hair must be dry.

• Don't be tempted to save on the cost of a touch-up of your relaxed hair by applying a straightening comb to the new growth. This is extremely damaging. You will be inviting trouble, and it will respond to your invitation in a way that might be irreversible!

• Don't pull the hair tightly as you straighten. This can result in traction and banded alopecia, which is a condition causing localized baldness.

• Don't be heavy-handed when applying hair grease prior to pressing.

THE NATURAL

The sixties and seventies were times that liberated our souls. "BLACK IS BEAUTI-FUL" was the new-found battle cry of millions of Blacks — women and men. These words reverberated through the halls of universities, churches and corporations. Black women shampooed their hair, and wore their hair naturally — with the pride and majesty of African queens. Free from hot combs, chemicals and other tools and products that seemed to hold them in bondage, Black women gleefully welcomed their new found liberty and unique form of self-expression and awareness.

While the natural is very easy to maintain, it, too, must be properly cared for and groomed. . . The first step to a beautiful natural (Afro) is an expert cut. Don't try to pat and force your Afro to succumb to a shape. Instead, go to a salon, and have your Afro shaped to compliment the shape of your face and features. To maintain your Afro, a trim every six weeks will help you achieve symmetry, balance and shape.

Your natural should be kept exceptionally clean and moisturized to add the sheen that is so very complimentary to this particular styling option. Shampoo with an oil-based shampoo, then condition hair. Add a small amount of lightweight hairdressing directly to the hair. Section hair and comb with a wide-toothed pick.

When your natural hair is dry, wet it a little before combing. The water will make combing easier; thereby, minimizing breakage. Use a natural boar bristle brush on your hair.

RELAX IT!

Relaxers have been improved greatly. Scientific improvements have resulted in hair that looks good — naturally. The new relaxers condition hair as they straighten. While many relaxers contain built-in conditioners, it is still of paramount importance that you condition your hair after you shampoo. Relaxers tend to deplete the hair of its natural moisture level. Intense moisturizing conditioners are recommended. Moisturizers are, in essence, state-of-the art conditioners, which will positively affect the balance of moisture in relaxed hair. Another product to try is a reconstructor, which fills in the areas of the hair that have been damaged through daily mishandling and abuse. The result is a shiny, radiant, smooth head of beautiful hair.

HOW DO RELAXERS (PERMS) ACTUALLY WORK?

The relaxer is a chemical process which permanently alters the natural structure of the hair. The relaxer chemically straightens the hair; while other perms chemically curl the hair. As the hair grows, a touch-up is necessary. The new growth will be of the same texture and curl pattern as the natural hair. When a touch-up is required, the stylist applies the relaxer to the new growth *only*. This enables the newly grown hair to match the straightened texture of the rest of the hair.

The dominant ingredient in relaxers is sodium hydroxide, commonly known as lye. Today the concentration of sodium hydroxide is usually two to three percent. This lower concentration has made relaxers gentler on the hair than relaxers of the past. The incident of breakage and hair loss has been greatly reduced, but the Black woman should not be lulled into a false sense of security. The process of applying a permanent relaxing solution to the hair is still a very dangerous one, and should be left in the hands of a highly skilled, trained and licensed hair care professional.

Petrolatum base is no longer necessary, thanks to the innovative, new formulas that have flooded the Black hair care market. One of the most creative and liberating innovations is the emulsion relaxer, which contains built-in moisturizers.

NO-LYE RELAXERS

According to Dr. Wesley S. Wilborn, an Atlanta dermatologist, the no-lye relaxer is a formula which does not contain sodium hydroxide. "The prototype no-lye is a mixture of guanidine carbonate and calcium hydroxide. When mixed together these two ingredients form guanidine hydroxide. The only chemical that is (correctly) called lye is sodium hydroxide." Dr. Wilborn adds that there are other hydroxides that are just as caustic as sodium hydroxide, where the net (adverse) effect on Black hair can be similar to lye. However, he does believe that guanidine hydroxide, which is the prototype, patented no-lye formula, is gentler on Black hair, but can be very drying. He suggests that the hair is given a good moisturizing treatment once-a-week, when a no-lye relaxer is used.

Finally, just because a relaxer is labeled "no-lye" doesn't mean that you can throw caution to the wind. This chemical, as with all chemicals, should be applied carefully. Follow the instructions and leave on for the prescribed amount of time to avoid damage to the hair. Dr. Wilborn says, "If you're getting your hair done with chemicals, try to choose someone who is competent. Most of the damage that is done by chemicals is done by the person who is applying it, and not by the chemical itself."

FADE TO BLACK

You might have noticed that your hair's natural color has faded since you started to relax your hair. This is because the sodium hydroxide contained in many relaxers tend to strip the hair of its natural color and moisture. Temporary or semipermanent hair color can be applied.

RELAXING AT HOME

While the chemical process of relaxing should be done by a professional hairstylist, there are many Black women who simply must relax at home -- either for convenience or economics. If you relax at home, read the instructions completely before proceeding. Follow the instructions explicitly to minimize possible damage to the hair and scalp.

Solicit the assistance of a friend or family member. No matter how skilled you might be in managing your own hair, the back of your head is going to be more than a challenge. Even if you're ambidextrous, a friend's extra set of hands and eyes will make all the difference in the world. Check with your hairstylist to see if your hair and scalp are in good enough condition to withstand chemical processing, and no matter how tempting, never give yourself a virginal perm (first-time relaxer). Additionally, a relaxer should never be applied on top of another chemical, i.e., curling process. Do not relax when you have permanent hair color, or you have recently removed braids or cornrows worn over a long period of time. If your scalp is scratched, irritated or damaged, wait until it is completely healed before undergoing this chemical process. All of these conditions warrant professional assistance.

Over-processing can result in localized hair loss, which can be irreversible.

Finally, if you can avoid relaxing your hair at home — do so. The money spent on having a professional apply the relaxer for you is money well spent. Remember, this is a *chemical* process, and it should be taken seriously. You can economize by shampooing, conditioning and styling your hair at home in-between touch-ups. Visit your stylist every six weeks (or longer) for a professional touch-up. Why? **BECAUSE YOU'RE WORTH IT!**

Relaxed hair is a wonderful styling option for Black women. An option that affords them styling diversity and versatility. One of the more popular methods of achieving many of these styles is the wet set (see Chapter 8). Use protein hair moisturizers containing glycerin and oil sheen sprays to give your relaxed hair a radiant shine.

SKIN PATCH AND STRAND TESTS

Before applying a relaxer, two tests should be administered. The first, a *skin patch test*, will determine whether you will have an allergic response to the chemicals contained in the relaxer. The second, *a strand test,* will determine how your hair will respond to the relaxer. Don't skip either of these tests.

THE CURLY PERMANENT

The curly permanent (perm) is another styling option available to the Black woman. To achieve this style, a two-step process is necessary. First, the hair is relaxed, rinsed and conditioned. A solution containing thioglycolates or bisulfites is, then, applied to the hair to alter its natural structure by breaking down the bonds of the hair. Hair is set on perming rods until the desired curl is achieved. The finished look is a halo of uniformed, luxurious curls. Longer hair will have a looser, cascading wave formation.

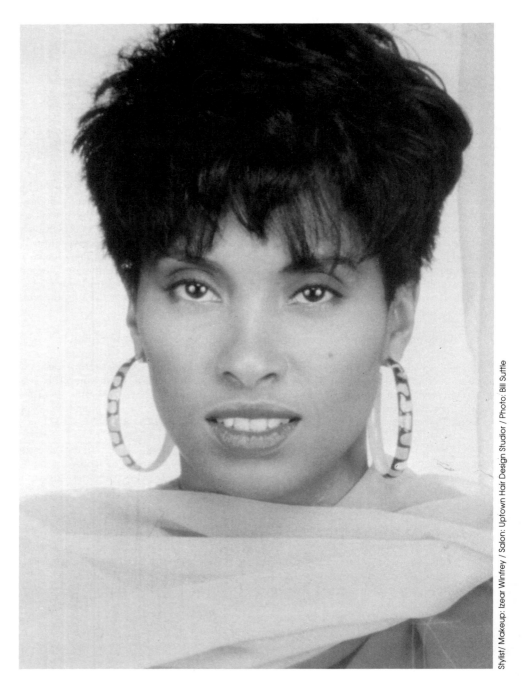

On The Cutting Edge

Stylist / Makeup: Izear Winfrey / Salon: Uptown Hair Design Studios / Photo: Bill Suttle

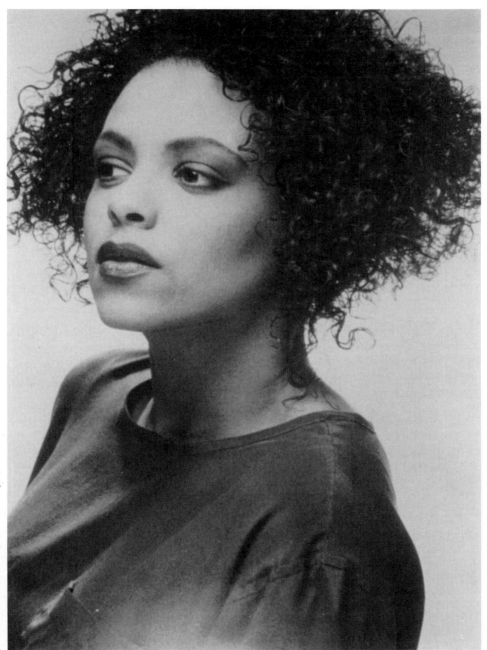

There Was A Little Girl With A Pretty Little Curl. . .

Curly perms thrive on moisture. Use moisturizers, activators and/or sheen spray products containing oils and glycerine several times daily. Moisture reactivates the curl. These products replenish the hair's natural moisture level and safeguard against breakage and split ends.

The curly perm is an excellent styling option for exercise-conscious and sports-minded Black women. The moisturizing products used for daily maintenance of the curl act as protectants against the drying effect of perspiration. Keep in mind, however, that regardless of whether your hair is relaxed, curled or natural, you should shampoo and condition it as soon as possible after working up a sweat.

Because there is less maintenance involved with the curly perm than the relaxer, there are fewer opportunities to traumatize the hair or cause breakage. The curly perm eliminates the need to roll the hair or to use curling irons. Dr. Gloria Campbell-D'Hue says that when this styling option is compatible to her patients' lifestyles, she recommends it. "All you have to do is shampoo and moisturize, and moisturization helps to coat the shaft of the hair. Hair is more supple (with the curl perm)," she advises.

Even with the many positive attributes of the curly perm, it is not without its drawbacks. The consequence of moisturizing the curl is often a very unbecoming "greasy kid look". Additionally, the dripping moisturizers often result in oil-stained upholstery, clothing and bed linen. USE ONLY AS MUCH MOISTURIZER AS IS NECESSARY TO MAINTAIN YOUR CURL. Don't overdo it.

Dermatologist Steven Thomas, M.D., says that it really doesn't matter which style his patients prefer. What does matter is how they take care of it. GOOD GROOMING PRACTICES AND MAINTENANCE ARE ESSENTIAL. "Hair care should not be oppressive, in terms of what it requires from you. It should be fairly simple. It should be routine, and it should not be something that is changed every two weeks, or everytime a new style becomes popular. You should find something that compliments you. Something that makes you feel comfortable, and at the same time, doesn't damage the hair. THE MOST IMPORTANT THING FOR HAIR IS DAMAGE CONTROL. Protect the hair from the environment and from abusive grooming and styling practices," he adds.

So, ladies, the choice is yours. If you would like to try a curly look, but the dripping wet-look turns you off, perhaps a texturizer is for you.

TEXTURIZERS

A texturizer is a milder version of the relaxer. With texturizers, the breakage of hair bonds is not as drastic, as in the relaxing process. The hair is therefore not as bone-straight as with a relaxer. Texturizers are not for everyone. The type of hair you have, the condition that it is in, and your lifestyle should be taken into consideration before undergoing the texturizing process. Texturized hair can offer you the opportunity of having the look of a curly perm, without the dripping moisturizers. It offers a more natural look. Afroesque styles can be achieved with a texturizer. (Afroesque is Afrocentric styling on hair that is mildly relaxed.)

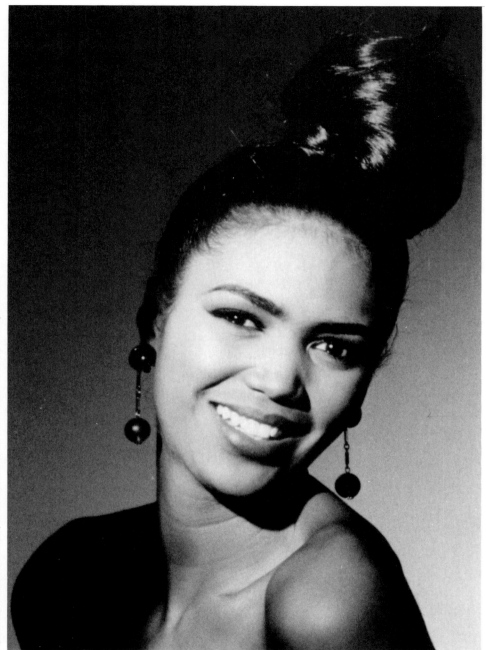

Tressed To Kill

BRAIDS AND CORNROWS

Cornrows are based in African tradition and continue to be a modern day expression of ethnic pride. They have the wonderful advantage of being carefree, and they last a very long time. You can even shampoo your hair without unbraiding it. You simply place a bit of shampoo into the palms of your hands and gently massage into the scalp and hair with the pads of your fingertips. After the shampoo, allow water to run freely through your hair. MAKE SURE YOU RINSE ALL TRACES OF SHAMPOO OUT OF YOUR HAIR. Wrapping your head, Turkish-style, blot excess water from the hair. To minimize frizziness and to maintain a sleek, smooth look, wrap your braids in a silky scarf. You can then go about the business of your day, allowing your hair to dry naturally. If you must leave the house, and simply do not have time to allow your hair to dry naturally, use a wide-nozzled blow dryer on a low temperature setting. Keep the dryer at least six inches from hair.

NEVER TOO TIGHT

Make sure that you do not braid your hair too tightly. This is extremely damaging. It's better to have to re-braid your hair more often, than to have no hair at all, which is exactly the circumstance that you will be facing. Braids worn too tightly will damage your hair and result in traction alopecia. All you have to do is look at some of the Black celebrities and public figures who have worn their hair braided tightly over a long period of time. Frontal loss is quite common with this hairstyle, if caution is not exercised. Don't let this discourage you from wearing this beautiful style, however. The rules are really quite simple: Don't braid too tightly, and don't wear braids for an extended period of time, without a bit of a rest in between.

Hold your head high, and step tall and proud with the regal bearing of an African queen, for that's what you are. Afrocentric hairstyling is a wonderful way of wearing your heart on your sleeve. It demonstrates pride in our rich African heritage. Your hair can be beautiful and make a strong cultural statement at the same time.

CHAPTER 16: To Dye Or Not To Dye

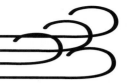

PIZZAZZ! PANACHE! SPIRIT! A dash and splash of color can be fun. Hair coloring offers diversity, versatility and excitement. There are basically three methods of getting color: rinse (temporary coloring), semipermanent and permanent.

COLOR ME BEAUTIFUL...

A woman's reason for choosing to dye her hair is as varied as the rainbow of shades she has to choose from. One woman might succumb to the seduction of television, magazines and advertisements to stay younger longer by opting to cover her grays. Another woman might choose to color her hair for adventure... Whatever your reason, if you opt to color, do so cautiously. There is really nothing difficult about coloring your hair, but as with any process, it should be approached intelligently. Many of the products on the market today are specifically designed for home use. Choose a product that is right for you and follow the directions.

One of the wonderful advantages of coloring one's hair is that the dye actually thickens the hair by coating the hair shaft. Permanent hair color swells the hair shaft as it is absorbed. This is a special bonus for women with thinning hair. As we age, many women's hair tend to thin. By coloring the hair, you're actually accomplishing two objectives with one process. First, you're getting rid of unwanted gray hair; and second, the consequence is thicker, fuller hair.

THE COLOR RINSE

A color rinse is a temporary, water soluble coloring, which lasts from shampoo-to-shampoo. Obviously, because of its lack of staying power, it allows you to be bold. You can venture into color palettes that you ordinarily wouldn't dream of applying to your hair. A bit of water and shampoo, and pouf! The color is gone. If you're really not sure about a particular color, use a rinse to experiment. If the result is good then you might try a more permanent dyeing solution.

THE SEMIPERMANENT COLOR

Semipermanent color does not contain peroxide or ammonia. The absence of these harsh chemical ingredients make semipermanent dyes a gentler and safer color option for Black women with relaxed or permed hair.

Semipermanent color coats, while permanent color penetrates the hair shaft. Dramatic hair color changes cannot be actualized effectively with semipermanent dyes. It will not lighten the hair, but it is actually quite effective at covering grays and intensifying the natural hair shade. Semipermanent color lasts from six to eight weeks.

VEGETABLE DYE — HENNA

Another form of semipermanent color is henna. Henna was touted as the natural way of obtaining color during the '80s. Henna is a natural vegetable dye, reddish in coloration. This method of coloring the hair goes all the way back to the days of Egyptian pyramids and Cleopatra. Black women with relaxers or curly perms should avoid henna. Henna will strip the hair of its natural oils and moisture, leaving it dry and brittle. After a couple of applications, the build-up of henna leaves hair with an unflattering orange cast. While henna does have properties that thicken the hair, after using henna, many women complain that they have difficulty getting a comb through their hair, and that it appears dull and lackluster.

The color obtained from henna will last from six to eight weeks.

JAZZING AND CELLOPHANE COLORS

The most common brand names of a relatively new type of semipermanent coloring (**hair glazes**) are Jazzing and Cellophane Colors. This exciting method of coloring the hair adds radiant shine, sheen and luxurious highlights to the hair. Glazes are comprised of food coloring and mica chips. The glaze is applied to the hair, and then the patron sits under a heat lamp for approximately thirty minutes. The heat from the lamp assists in the absorption of the solution.

Glazes can be used safely on chemically processed hair and last from four to six weeks.

PERMANENT COLOR

Permanent coloring is best left to Black women with natural hair. The inclusion of peroxide and ammonia in permanent dyes makes them too harsh for processed hair. While some Black women with relaxed hair have had success with permanent dyes, a far greater number have met with disastrous results. If your hair has been relaxed, curled, or in any way chemically treated, steer clear of permanent dyes!

Even Black women with virginal hair should leave the permanent coloring job to the skilled hands of a trained hairstylist or colorist. Permanent dyes will alter the structure of your hair. It's a two-step process: First, it strips your natural hair color; and second, it recolors the hair. The peroxide contained in permanent hair coloring swells the hair shaft as it penetrates. This swelling process robs the hair of its elasticity, leaving it extremely vulnerable to breakage. On the other hand, this swelling also makes the hair look fuller, thicker and more voluminous.

Permanent coloring of the hair is serious business. A professional stylist or colorist can evaluate whether this process is right for you, and then, apply it properly.

THE SKIN PATCH TEST

Semipermanent and permanent coloring *always* require a skin patch test. This test will ascertain whether you will have an allergic reaction to the chemicals contained in the hair coloring product. The test should be conducted 24 hours prior to use.

THE STRAND TEST

While the skin patch test evaluates your *skin's* sensitivity to the chemicals contained in the dye, a strand test will determine how your *hair* will react to the chemicals.

A WORD TO THE WISE

Coloring the hair is indeed a momentous occasion, and one that should be given serious deliberation. Coloring actually affects the composition and structure of the hair. Proceed with caution and intelligence. RINSE HAIR THOROUGHLY and follow-through with a moisturizing conditioner.

COLOR SELECTION

Try not to stray too far away from your natural coloring as a Black woman. Is blond really right for you? If you're toying with the idea of finding out first-hand whether blondes really do have more fun, try one of the wash-out color sprays to see if such a drastic change is realistic, or if it's really what you want. Choose a color that is complimentary to your skin tone. One that enhances your natural beauty.

CHAPTER 17: Fun In The Sun With Colored And Chemically-Treated Hair

BERMUDA! TOBAGO! JAMAICA! THE BAHAMAS!

You've worked all year. . . kicking, jumping, flexing and sweating with "the Fonda" and other exercise gurus, and it hasn't been for naught. YOU LOOK MARVELOUS! That white bikini is really saying something, as it caresses your sumptuous curves and waves. You've followed the instructions in this handbook, and your hair is healthy, beautiful and turning heads. You just can't wait to strut your stuff along the pink sands of your favorite island get-away. BUT WAIT.... Before diving into that Olympic-sized hotel swimming pool or the ocean, make sure that you take a few precautionary measures to safeguard your colored or chemically-treated hair against the harmful effects of chlorine, ocean minerals and the drying rays of the sun.

Coat your hair with an oil-rich conditioner that contains a sunscreen. It will serve as a protectant against the elements. Always wear a properly fitted swimming cap before going into the water. To rid your hair of chlorine or the ocean's damaging minerals, rinse your hair thoroughly after swimming. When you get back to the hotel room, shampoo. Chlorine is extremely harmful to all hair (white and Black). It will strip your hair color. If you have a semipermanent dye in your hair, you should wait a couple of weeks before diving in, or the color will run down your face.

Wear a sexy hat or silky, feminine scarf to protect your relaxed or permed hair from the drying effects of the sun. Have a ball, but don't throw caution to the wind. After all, there is life after your vacation, and you don't want to ruin your hair for eight days and seven nights under the sun.

It only takes a minute of thought and common sense to safeguard your glorious locks against damage.

BON VOYAGE!

CHAPTER 18: Fabulous Fakes!

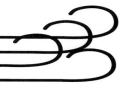

ALL TRESSED UP!

Flair! Versatility! Diversity! By simply adding a wig, fall, chignon, ponytail, braid or switch, you can change your look dramatically. The construction of wigs and hairpieces is better than ever. People have worn wigs from the beginning of time (both men and women). The new lighter weight designs make wigs more comfortable to wear today than in the past. Synthetic wigs and hairpieces are also mimicking the texture and curl pattern of Black hair with much greater accuracy today.

HAIR-RAISING TALES

"Rapunzel, Rapunzel, let down your hair." And, she did —literally. These words were spoken in a fairytale which relays a tale of a damsel in distress, who lowers her long, blond braid out of a castle window, where she is being held captive. Her knight in shining armor shimmies up her hair (using it as a rope) and rescues the fair damsel. Of course, they lived happily ever after.

Black women are barraged by images of women with long, flowing hair from the time they are little girls. As children, their fairytale books and dolls foster the wonders of long locks. As they get **older** , magazines, films, MTV, and yes, even BET, step in and continue to reinforce this concept. In actuality, there are very few women (white or Black) with Rapunzel length hair.

Black women have long had a love affair with "fabulous fakes", whether it is weaved hair, extensions, falls, pieces, switches or wigs. Many Black women have also mastered the technique of making these store-bought items look convincingly real. Only their hairstylist knows for sure.

Wigs, weaves, hairpieces . . . They're fun! They can add diversity to your look, and they're convenient. As long as you don't enslave yourself to them, but rather, use them as a fashion accessory, there really isn't anything terribly wrong with them. Don't neglect your natural hair while wearing them, however.

HAIRWEAVING

We have witnessed an ever-increasing popularity in hairweaving during the late '80s and early '90s. Everywhere you look, you see a sister tossing a long lock of weaved hair over her shoulder. Many Black comedians have picked-up on this trend, and are using it as material in their stand-up routines. This time around, white women have also gotten into the act. They have picked up on the wonders of weaving and are using this technique to add length, volume and dimension to their own hair.

When the fake hair is selected carefully to match the color and texture of the natural hair, weaves can be extremely realistic. There are three methods of weaving — needle and thread, braiding and bonding.

According to Dr. Steve Thomas, the hairweaving process has improved greatly. He says that he is seeing fewer patients with hair problems that are associated with weaving. "The adverse effects that I use to see quite frequently have diminished greatly," he says.

TIME-SAVERS

If you're running short on time, and need the time-saving convenience of a wig or chignon — fine. Whatever you do, don't use wigs, hairpieces and weaves on an on-going, consistent basis. Your natural hair should be cared for and allowed to breathe freely without the weight of a wig suffocating your scalp. If you wear a wig, make sure that you keep the wig clean, and don't neglect your own hair. A wig cap will help to safeguard your natural hair from undue friction.

Some really wonderful looks can be achieved with hairpieces... ranging from cute-as-a-button, bouncy ponytails to sophisticated, elegant chignons for black-tie affairs. The one thing that must be kept in mind is that every cute, store-bought ponytail and chignon has to be pinned to your real hair, and therein lies the problem. The constant pinning in the same location, and tight pulling of your hair to **accommodate** the hairpiece, can result in traction alopecia (hair loss).

While there are positive attributes to fake hair, there is nothing like the real thing. If you take care of your natural hair, you just might find that you won't want to wear fake hair as much and probably not at all.

AIN'T NOTHING LIKE THE REAL THING?

While many Black women adore fake hair, an article appearing in the November, 1991 issue of *Essence* magazine, written by Elsie B. Washington, discovered that Black men have a distinct aversion to fake hair. One Black man quoted in the article, said: "Hate extensions." Another said: "Hate weaves." And still another said: "Work with what you have, rather than covering it up dramatically. I appreciate women who accentuate the beauty of their natural hair."

According to a rebuttal article appearing in the May 1992 issue of *Essence* magazine, sisters responded to the brothers' November advice by saying: "We love you brothers, but please stay outta our hair." Sisters, responding to the November article, felt overwhelmingly that they (and they alone) had the right to define themselves for themselves, and that the way they chose to wear their hair was an inherent and integral aspect of that definition of self. It's our choice!

THE FINAL WORD

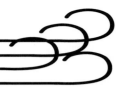

I saw her yesterday. She sauntered... She swayed... She sashayed... She pranced. Her large, luminous eyes perched precariously on high chiseled cheekbones. Her skin was mocha sprinkled with cinnamon.

When she moved her hair danced, forming a halo of energy around her head. It giggled... It laughed... It talked... It shouted. Her hair had a big mouth. It cried: "Look at me. I'm beautiful!" It beckoned me closer. I wanted to touch it. So rich... So soft... So bouncy. It seemed to have a mind of its own. It was the hair of a woman who cared. It was the hair of a woman who had made a commitment. It was the hair of a Black woman who knew that GOOD HAIR IS HEALTHY HAIR! That woman can be you. COMMITMENT...THAT'S ALL IT TAKES, AND A CELEBRATION OF SELF.

INDEX

☐ YES! I would like additional copies of **BLACK HAIR IS. . .**
The Complete Hair Care Guide For Today's Black Woman

QUANTITY

_____ **BLACK HAIR IS,** Marilyn Singleton, $14.95

Please add $1.00 postage and handling for one book; 50¢ for each additional book. Georgia residents add sales tax.

Print or type name and address clearly:

Name: _____

Address: _____ Apt. _____

City: _____ State: _____ Zip: _____

Send check or money order to:

IMAGE PERFECT COMMUNICATIONS, INC.
1480 F Terrell Mill Road
Suite 289
Marietta, GA 30067